Y. ALLOW

Get Lean and Trim Without Going To the Gym

15 Bodyweight Exercises You Can Do At Home

This book was professionally typeset on Reedsy.
Find out more at reedsy.com

Contents

I

Get Lean and Trim Without Going To the Gym

Introduction

Why pay money to go to a gym when you can get lean and trim at home? This short book aims to give you a bunch of exercises you can perform in the comfort of your own home without an expensive gym membership or gym equipment. The exercises listed within use only your body weight and can be combined in whatever way suits you to create a solid workout routine which will help you achieve your fitness goals. You can add weights or resistance bands if you have them, but they are unnecessary. Common household items such as a bottle of water or a tin of beans can be used to add resistance if you want to.

The book is split up into three main sections:

- Cardio / Full Body Exercises
- Core / Upper Body Exercises
- Legs / Lower Body Exercises

All exercises can be performed as either repetitions (reps, usually 6–10) or for a set amount of time, e.g., 30 seconds. The Cardiovascular (Cardio) exercises lend themselves better to the latter and can also serve as warm-up exercises, but do whatever feels most comfortable for you.

Before getting started, let's talk about safety.

Always consider the various safety aspects of the exercise and your environment to ensure a safe and successful fitness journey. If you have any existing health conditions or concerns, please consult with a healthcare professional.

Start gently to warm up and increase blood flow to muscles, preparing the body for more strenuous activity. Similarly, at the end of your workout, include some cool-down exercises to bring your heart rate and breathing back to normal. Cardio exercises suited to warm-ups and cool-downs are marked on the relevant pages in this book. Stretching is also highly advisable, along with some deep breathing, both to reduce muscle soreness and improve overall flexibility.

Listen to your body. These exercises should not cause pain or severe discomfort. Please stop if you experience any such symptoms. Make sure you allow sufficient time to recover between exercises as needed. Rest days are as important as exercise days.

Do not try and progress too quickly. Some exercises will be more challenging than others. The goal should be to make a little bit of progress at a time. For example, you may only be able to manage two push-ups. That's OK. Over time, you will be able to do many more. Your fitness journey should be thought of more like a marathon than a sprint.

Safety is important! Keeping it in mind will help make your workouts more effective and promote a healthy and sustainable approach towards any physical activity. I wish you well as you embark on your fitness journey.

How to use this book – A Blueprint

To get the most out of this book, I would encourage you to follow a High-Intensity Interval Training (HIIT) approach. This involves alternating between short, intense bursts of exercise and short reset periods. For example, 30 seconds of *"give it everything you've got"*, followed by 30 seconds of recovery (or perhaps a 40/20 split) for two or three sets. The intensity can be dialled up or down depending on your own fitness levels/goals.

Benefits of following this approach include improved cardiovascular health, improved oxygen consumption, increased metabolism, efficient fat-burning, preservation of lean muscle mass and it is very time efficient.Workouts can take as little as 15 minutes (not including the warm-up, and cool-down elements) if you're short on time and still provide quick and impactful results, far exceeding that of a traditional 30-minute cardio workout. Below are two examples of a HIIT workout.

Workout #1 – 15 minutes

- 60 secs Jumping Jacks followed by 20 secs rest.
  Repeat twice more.
- 30 secs plank followed by 30 secs rest.
  Repeat once.

- 60 secs body weight squats followed by 20 secs rest.
  Repeat twice more.
- 30 secs push-ups followed by 30 secs rest.
  Repeat once.
- 45 secs Squat Jumps followed by 15 secs rest.
  Repeat twice more.

Workout #2 – 20 minutes

- 60 secs Jumping Jacks followed by 20 secs rest.
  Repeat twice more.
- 30 secs Wall Sits followed by 30 secs rest.
  Repeat twice more.
- 40 secs Body weight Squats followed by 20 secs rest.
  Repeat twice more.
- 60 secs Running on the Spot followed by 30 secs rest.
  Repeat twice more.
- 30 secs Reverse Crunches followed by 30 secs rest.
  Repeat twice more.
- 40 secs Burpees followed by 10 secs rest.
  Repeat.

Utilise a stopwatch to keep time, or choose from a plethora of free (or paid) HIIT apps, available on both Android and iPhone platforms.

II

Cardio/Full Body Exercises

Cardio exercises offer a range of benefits. These include strengthening your heart, increased lung capacity, increased calorie burn, increased stamina and energy levels, better sleep and sharper focus to name a few. They also release endorphins (the body's happy hormone) into the bloodstream, making you feel better. Cardio exercises are also great for warming up the body before more intense workouts and cooling down after them as they tend to target multiple areas of the body.

Jumping Jacks

A great, low-impact way to get your heart rate up and engage multiple muscle groups. They are a simple but effective exercise that boosts heart health, improves coordination and endurance, and can serve as a dynamic warm-up, preparing the body for more intense activity by increasing blood flow to all major muscle groups. They can also contribute to increased calorie burn.

Muscles engaged:

- Cardiovascular system
- Calves
- Quadriceps and Hamstrings (front and back thigh muscles)
- Hip Flexors
- Abdominals and obliques (core muscles)
- Back muscles
- Triceps and deltoids (arms and shoulder muscles)

Starting Position

- Stand with your feet together and arms at your sides.

Begin the Exercise

- Jump and simultaneously spread your legs shoulder-width apart.
- Raise your arms overhead, forming an "X" shape with your body.

Return to Starting Position

- Jump again, bringing your feet back together and lowering your arms to your sides.
- Land softly to absorb impact and protect your joints.

Repetition

- Repeat the sequence at a brisk, rhythmic pace.

Breathing

- Inhale as you spread your legs and raise your arms.
- Exhale as they return to the starting position.

Tips on Good Form

- Keep your core engaged (by pulling your belly button to your spine) to stabilize your body.
- Land softly with slightly bent knees to minimize impact on joints.
- Maintain a steady and controlled pace.

Challenging?

- If the impact is too intense, consider doing a low-impact version by stepping one foot out to the side at a time while raising your arms.

Duration

- Perform them for anywhere upwards of 30 seconds, based on your fitness level and workout goals.

Running on the Spot

Another simple, effective, warm-up exercise to get the heart rate up and increase overall endurance. Multiple muscle groups are engaged, leading to better agility and coordination, and as with most of the exercises in this book, can be performed anywhere.

Muscles engaged:

- Cardiovascular system
- Calves
- Quadriceps and hamstrings (front and back thigh muscles)
- Hip Flexors
- Abdominals and obliques (core muscles)
- Back muscles
- Triceps and deltoids (arms and shoulder muscles)

Starting Position

- Stand tall with your feet hip-width apart.
- Keep your shoulders relaxed, and maintain good posture with your chest up and core engaged (by pulling your belly button towards your spine).

Begin the Exercise

- Lift your knees alternately towards your chest in a marching or jogging motion.
- Coordinate your arm movements with your legs, as you would when running.
- Swing your arms naturally, bent at the elbows, in rhythm with your leg movements.
- Land lightly on the balls of your feet with each step.
- Avoid heavy stomping, and maintain a quick and light pace.

Repetition

- Continue alternating your arm and leg movements at a comfortable pace.

Breathing

- Breathe naturally and rhythmically.
- Inhale and exhale steadily to support the increased heart rate.

Tips on Good Form

- Keep your core muscles engaged throughout the exercise.
- This helps to stabilize your body making the workout more effective.

Challenging?

- Try lifting your knees higher for more of a challenge.

Duration:

- Perform this exercise for a set duration, upwards of 60 seconds, depending on your fitness level and workout goals.

Burpees

An efficient and effective, full-body exercise that targets multiple muscle groups and boosts both strength and cardiovascular endurance. They are made of a combination of exercises, a squat, plank and jump, rolled into one. They can also be used as a warm-up exercise; depending on your fitness level, you might prefer to warm up *before* attempting them.

Muscles engaged:

- Cardiovascular system
- Calves
- Quadriceps and hamstrings (front and back thigh muscles)
- Hip Flexors
- Abdominals and obliques (core muscles)
- Back muscles
- Pectoral and deltoids (chest and shoulders)
- Triceps (back of upper arms)

Starting Position

- Begin in a standing position with your feet shoulder-width apart.
- Maintain a straight posture with your shoulders back and chest up.

Begin the Exercise

- Lower your body into a squat position by bending your knees and bringing your hands to the ground.
- Jump your feet back, landing in a plank (*see page 27*) position.
- Ensure your body forms a straight line from head to heels.
- Jump your feet back towards your hands, returning to the squat position.
- Maintain a strong core and keep your weight on your heels.
- Explosively jump into the air, reaching your arms overhead.
- Fully extend your body at the top of the jump.
- Land softly on the balls of your feet to absorb the impact.

Repetition

- Immediately go into the next repetition.
- Perform burpees continuously for a set duration or a specific number of repetitions.

Breathing

- Breathe naturally and rhythmically.
- Inhale and exhale steadily to support the increased heart rate.

Tips on Good Form

- Keep a steady and controlled rhythm to ensure proper form and reduce the risk of injury.
- Tighten your core muscles throughout the movement to provide stability and protect your lower back.

Challenging?

- If the standard burpee is too challenging, try stepping back instead of jumping.
- For more of a challenge, add a push-up (*see page 30*) after landing in the plank position (keeping your elbows close to your body), or add a Jumping Jack at the top of the movement.

Duration

- Perform this exercise for a set duration, or a specific number of reps, depending on your fitness level and workout goals.

Mountain Climbers

Mountain climbers are a dynamic and effective full-body exercise that engages multiple muscle groups, including the core, arms, and legs. They provide a solid cardiovascular challenge while targeting core strength and stability.

Muscles engaged:

- Cardiovascular system
- Quadriceps and hamstrings (front and back thigh muscles)
- Hip Flexors
- Abdominals and obliques (core muscles)
- Back muscles
- Pectoral and deltoids (chest and shoulders)
- Triceps (back of upper arms)

Starting Position

- Begin in a plank (*see page 27*) position with your hands directly beneath your shoulders.
- Ensure your body forms a straight line from your head to your heels.
- Engage your core muscles by pulling your belly button toward your

spine.
- Keep your shoulders stabilized and your wrists aligned with your shoulders.

Begin the Exercise

- Lift your right knee towards your chest while keeping your left leg extended.
- Aim to bring your knee as close to your chest as possible.
- Quickly switch legs by bringing your right leg back to the plank position while simultaneously bringing your left knee towards your chest.

Repetition

- Continue alternating legs in a running motion, mimicking the movement of running on the spot.
- Perform mountain climbers for a set duration or a specific number of repetitions, depending on your fitness level.

Breathing

- Coordinate your breathing with the movement. Inhale and exhale in a steady rhythm to support your cardiovascular system.

Tips on Good Form

- Keep your hips low and stable throughout the exercise.
- Avoid letting your hips rise or sag, maintaining a plank position.
- Maintain a controlled and steady pace to ensure proper form and engagement of the targeted muscles.

Challenging?

- If the standard mountain climber is too challenging, perform a modified version by bringing one knee at a time towards your chest.
- For more of a challenge, increase the intensity by speeding up the movement, or bringing each knee towards the opposite elbow to engage the obliques, but always prioritize maintaining good form.

Duration

- Perform this exercise for a set duration, or a specific number of reps, depending on your fitness level and workout goals.

Bear Crawls

Bear crawls are a dynamic and full-body exercise engaging multiple muscle groups, including the core, shoulders, and legs. They are functional, and versatile, promote core stability, enhance coordination, and do provide a full-body workout.

Muscles engaged:

- Abdominals and obliques (core muscles)
- Deltoids (shoulder muscles)
- Back muscles
- Quadriceps and hamstrings (front and back thigh muscles)
- Biceps and triceps (front and back upper arm muscles)
- Hip Flexors
- Forearm muscles

Starting Position

- Begin on your hands and knees on a mat or a soft surface.
- Ensure your wrists are directly under your shoulders, and your knees are under your hips.
- Lift your knees slightly off the ground, creating a hover position.
- Your weight should be evenly distributed between your hands and

toes.

Begin the Exercise

- Start crawling forward by moving your right hand and left foot simultaneously.
- Follow with your left hand and right foot to maintain balance.
- Continue moving in a coordinated fashion, mimicking a crawling motion.
- Keep your movements controlled and deliberate.
- Avoid letting your knees touch the ground.
- Engage your core muscles to stabilize your body as you move.
- Keep your back straight and avoid rounding or arching.
- Your body should form a straight line from your head to your heels.

Repetition

- Continue crawling forward for a set distance or duration.
- To crawl backwards, reverse the movement by moving your left hand and right foot, followed by your right hand and left foot.
- Perform bear crawls for a set number of reps or a specific distance.
- Gradually increase the intensity and duration as you become more comfortable with the movement.

Breathing

- Breathe naturally, maintaining a steady breathing pattern throughout the bear crawl.

Tips on Good Form

- Keep your body low to the ground, maintaining a hover position with knees off the ground for optimal engagement.
- Focus on controlled and intentional movements to maximize the effectiveness of the exercise.

Challenging?

- If these bear crawls are too challenging, try moving from side to side, one limb at a time.
- For a more challenging exercise, try moving forwards and backwards in a circle, or simply increasing the duration of the crawl.

Duration

- Perform this exercise for a set duration, or a set distance, depending on your fitness level and workout goals.

III

Core/Upper Body Exercises

I like to call these confidence-boosting exercises. Your core and upper body are the most noticeable muscle groups when it comes to achieving that lean, trim look. Here are five exercises that will assist you in getting there.

Plank

Plank

This is a deceptively simple, yet very effective exercise for building a powerful midsection. It can build endurance, stabilize your spine, and build the strength needed to stabilise your body through various other activities.

Muscles engaged:

- Abdominals and obliques (core muscles).
- Back muscles.
- Glutes and hip flexors.
- Deltoids and trapezius (shoulders and upper back).
- Triceps (back of upper arms).
- Quadriceps and hamstrings (front and back thigh muscles).

Starting Position

- Begin on a mat or a flat surface, facing the ground.
- Position your hands directly beneath your shoulders, palms facing down.
- Extend your legs straight out, toes pointing down.

Body Alignment

- Keep your body in a straight line from your head to your heels. Engage your core muscles by pulling your belly button towards your spine.
- Ensure your shoulders are directly above your wrists.
- Maintain a neutral neck position by looking down at the ground.
- Avoid arching your neck up or letting it droop down.
- Squeeze your glutes to keep your hips in line with your back.
- Make sure your legs are straight, with a slight tension in your quadriceps.

Repetition

- Hold the plank position for as long as you can, gradually increasing the duration as your strength improves.

Breathing

- Inhale and exhale deeply, maintaining steady breath throughout the exercise.

Tips on Good Form

- Don't let your hips sag or lift too high; maintain a straight line.
- Avoid rounding or arching your back; engage your core muscles to keep a flat spine.
- If you prefer, you can perform a forearm plank by lowering onto your forearms.
- Elbows should be directly beneath your shoulders.

Challenging?

- If you find the full plank challenging, start with a modified version by keeping your knees on the ground.

Duration

- Perform this exercise for as long as possible without sacrificing form.

Push-Ups

Performing push-ups is an effective bodyweight exercise that strengthens the chest, shoulders, triceps, and core. They are very versatile and can be adapted to various fitness levels. Consistent practice will not only strengthen your upper body but also enhance overall muscular endurance.

Muscles engaged:

- Pectorals (chest)
- Deltoids (shoulders)
- Triceps (back of upper arms)
- Abdominals and obliques (core muscles)
- Back muscles
- Glutes and hip flexors
- Rhomboids and trapezius (shoulder blades and upper back)
- Quadriceps and hamstrings (front and back thigh muscles)

Starting Position

- Begin in a plank (*see page 27*) position with your hands placed slightly wider than shoulder-width apart.
- Position your hands firmly on the ground, fingers pointing forward

or slightly turned outward.

- Keep your elbows close to your body at a 45-degree angle.
- Engage your core by tightening your abdominal muscles.
- Ensure your body forms a straight line from head to heels.

Begin the Exercise

- Lower your body towards the ground by bending your elbows.
- Keep your body in a straight line; don't allow your hips to sag or push up.
- Lower your chest until it almost touches the ground or hovers just above it.
- Ensure a full range of motion without compromising form.

Return to Starting Position

- Push through your palms to straighten your arms and return to the starting position.
- Fully extend your elbows at the top of the movement.

Repetition

- Perform the desired number of repetitions, maintaining proper form throughout.

Breathing

- Inhale as you lower your body.
- Exhale as you push back up to the starting position.

Tips on Good Form

- Distribute your weight evenly between your hands.
- Avoid letting your elbows flare out.
- Maintain a straight line from your head to your heels throughout the movement.

Challenging?

- If traditional push-ups are challenging, start with knee push-ups or incline push-ups against a sturdy surface such as a chair or table. Maintain that straight line from your head to either your knees or heels depending on which version you go for.
- For more of a challenge, try bringing your hands closer together.

Duration

- Perform this exercise for a set duration, or a specific number of reps, depending on your fitness level and workout goals.

Tricep Dips

A great exercise for strengthening the triceps and engaging multiple upper-body muscle groups to support the movement and maintain stability. They effectively target the triceps, helping to strengthen and tone the back of your arms and can be done almost anywhere.

Muscles engaged:

- Triceps (back of upper arms)
- Anterior deltoids (front part of the shoulders)
- Pectorals (chest)
- Rhomboids and trapezius (shoulder blades and upper back)
- Abdominals and obliques (core muscles)
- Back muscles
- Forearms

Starting Position

- Find a sturdy chair, or the edge of a countertop no more than waist-high.
- Ensure the surface is stable and can support your body weight.
- Stand facing away from the chosen surface and place your hands on the surface, shoulder-width apart, with your fingers pointing

forward.

- Keep your wrists straight and your hands firmly gripping the surface edge.
- Walk your feet forward a few steps, extending your legs in front of you.
- Keep your heels on the ground, creating a slight bend in your knees.
- Your body should be in a straight line with your arms fully extended.

Begin the Exercise

- Lower your body by bending your elbows, allowing them to flare out to the sides.
- Lower until your upper arms are parallel to the ground or slightly below.
- Aim to keep your elbows at a 90-degree angle, forming an L-shape with your arms.

Return to Starting Position

- Push through your palms to straighten your arms and return to the starting position.
- Fully extend your elbows at the top of the movement.

Repetition

- Perform the desired number of repetitions, maintaining proper form throughout.

Breathing

- Inhale as you lower your body.

- Exhale as you push back up to the starting position.

Tips on Good Form

- Perform the exercise with controlled movements to engage the triceps effectively.
- Keep your shoulders down and away from your ears to avoid unnecessary strain.

Challenging?

- If the full tricep dip is too challenging, bend your knees more to reduce the load on your triceps by using a lower stable surface, such as a bench or chair.
- For more of a challenge, lift one leg off the ground and engage your core by pulling your belly button to your spine.

Duration

- Perform this exercise for a set duration, or a specific number of reps, depending on your fitness level and workout goals.

Dumbbell Rows

Dumbbell rows are an effective compound exercise that targets the muscles in your upper back. Dumbbell rows are a great addition to your back workout routine, helping to strengthen and sculpt the muscles in your upper back. Include them for a well-rounded back training session.

Muscles engaged:

- Latissimus dorsi (lats – largest back muscle)
- Rhomboids and trapezius (shoulder blades and upper back)
- Posterior deltoids (rear part of the shoulders)
- Biceps (front of the upper arm)
- Forearm muscles

Starting Position

- If you have dumbbells, great! If not, a bottle of water or even a tin of beans will do. You'll also need a flat bench or a couple of chairs for support.
- Stand with your feet shoulder-width apart.
- Hold a dumbbell (or other object) in your left hand with a neutral grip (palm facing your body).

- Line up the chairs and place your right knee on one and your right hand on the other, or use a bench if you have one.
- Your left foot should be on the ground, creating a stable base.
- Ensure your back is straight, forming a parallel line with the ground.
- Your left hand with the weight should be hanging directly below your left shoulder.

Begin the Exercise

- Pull the weight in your left hand towards your hip by bending your elbow.
- Keep your elbow close to your body and your upper arm parallel to the ground.
- At the top of the movement, squeeze your shoulder blades together to engage the muscles in your upper back.

Return to Starting Position

- Lower the weight in a controlled manner until your arm is fully extended.
- Maintain tension in your back muscles throughout the entire range of motion.

Repetition

- Perform the desired number of repetitions before switching sides by placing your left knee and left hand on the bench and rowing with your right hand.

Breathing

- Exhale as you lift the weight.
- Inhale as you lower it back down.

Tips on Good Form

- Keep your back straight, and your neck in a neutral position throughout the exercise.
- Maintain a stable base with the knee and hand on the bench and the opposite foot on the ground.
- Ensure a full range of motion by extending your arm fully at the bottom and squeezing your shoulder blades at the top.

Duration

- Perform this exercise for a set duration, or a specific number of reps on each arm, depending on your fitness level and workout goals.

Leg Raises

A fantastic isolation exercise for strengthening and toning the lower abdominal muscles and increasing overall core strength. They also engage other muscle groups for stability and support.

Muscles engaged:

- Abdominals and obliques (core muscles)
- Hip flexors (muscles at the front of the hips)
- Lower back
- Quadriceps (front thigh muscles)
- Hip Adductors (muscles on the inner thigh)

Starting Position

- Lie flat on your back on a mat or the floor.
- Place your hands either under your glutes or at your sides for support.

Begin the Exercise

- Lift your legs off the ground.
- Use your abdominal muscles to lift your legs, keeping them straight

and ensuring a controlled and deliberate movement.

- Aim to raise them vertically towards the ceiling without using momentum or swinging them.
- Lift your hips slightly off the ground at the top of the movement to engage the lower abdominal muscles more effectively.
- Hold the raised position for a moment, focusing on squeezing your lower abs.

Return to Starting Position

- Lower your legs back down to just above the ground in a controlled manner.
- Avoid letting your feet touch the ground between repetitions.

Repetition

- Perform the desired number of repetitions, maintaining proper form throughout.

Breathing

- Exhale as you lift your legs.
- Inhale as you lower them back down.

Tips on Good Form

- Keep your back flat on the ground throughout the exercise to avoid arching.
- Tighten your core to stabilize your lower back and maximize the effectiveness of the exercise.
- The lowering phase is crucial. Lower your legs slowly and with

control to engage the muscles effectively.

Challenging?

- If straight leg raises are challenging, you can perform the exercise with your knees slightly bent.
- Another, easier variation of this exercise is the seated leg raise. Sit upright on a chair and take turns raising each leg straight out in front of you to hip height (or as high as you can manage).

Duration

- Perform this exercise for a set duration, or a specific number of reps, depending on your fitness level and workout goals.

IV

Legs/Lower Body Exercises

Lower body exercises have so many health benefits. They engage the stabilizing muscles to enhance balance and coordination. They improve functional fitness for basic daily tasks such as lifting objects, climbing stairs, or even just walking. Additionally, strengthening the muscles in the thighs, hips and lower back can contribute to having better posture, reducing the risk of back pain and discomfort.

Lunges

Performing lunges is an effective exercise for targeting the muscles in your legs and glutes while also engaging your core for stability. They target various muscle groups simultaneously, support functional movement patterns, and can be performed either forward or backward.

Muscles engaged:

- Quadriceps and hamstrings (front and back thigh muscles)
- Glutes
- Adductors (inner thigh muscles)
- Calves
- Back muscles
- Abdominals (core muscles)
- Hip flexors (muscles at the front of the hips)

Starting Position

- Stand with your feet hip-width apart, hands on your hips or at your sides.

Begin the Exercise

- Take a step forward (forward lunge) with your right foot, ensuring a stride length that allows both knees to bend at a 90-degree angle.
- For the reverse lunge, take a step backwards.
- Bend both knees simultaneously, lowering your body towards the ground.
- Ensure your front knee is directly above your ankle, and your back knee hovers just above the floor.
- Keep your torso upright, shoulders back, and chest lifted.
- Engage your core muscles to maintain balance.

Return to Starting Position

- Push through your front heel to return to the starting position.
- Bring your right foot back beside your left.

Repetition

- Repeat the movement with your left leg, alternating between legs for each repetition.

Tips on Good Form

- Ensure your knees track over your toes, avoiding inward collapse.
- Maintain an upright posture to engage the correct muscles and prevent strain on your lower back.
- Perform lunges with controlled movements to enhance effectiveness and reduce the risk of injury.

Challenging?

- For more of a challenge, you could try performing lunges while

walking forward, alternating legs with each step.
- Another challenge could be to add a knee lift when returning to the starting position to engage your core further.

Duration

- Perform this exercise for a set duration, or a specific number of reps, depending on your fitness level and workout goals.

Wall Sits

An excellent isometric exercise that targets the muscles in your thighs, for building lower body strength. Include them in your lower body workout routine to improve muscular endurance and overall leg strength.

Muscles engaged:

- Quadriceps and hamstrings (front and back thigh muscles)
- Glutes
- Adductors (inner thigh muscles)
- Calves
- Back muscles
- Abdominals (core muscles)

Starting Position

- Find a clear wall and stand with your back against it.
- Place your feet about hip-width apart, and step forward a few inches from the wall.

Begin the Exercise

- Slide your back down the wall while bending your knees, and keep your entire back against the wall, with your shoulders and head touching.
- Lower your body until your thighs are parallel to the ground.
- Ensure your knees are directly above your ankles, forming a 90-degree angle.
- Your heels should remain about hip-width apart and a comfortable distance away from the wall.
- Ensure your knees are aligned with your toes and not collapsing inward.
- Distribute your weight evenly through your heels and the balls of your feet.
- Aim to have your thighs parallel to the ground, creating a right angle at your knees.

Repetition

- Hold the wall sit position for as long as you can maintain proper form.

Breathing

- Breathe naturally and avoid holding your breath during the wall sit.
- Inhale and exhale in a controlled manner.

Tips on Good Form

- Keep your back flat against the wall and avoid arching or rounding your back, keeping it flat against the wall.
- Tighten your core to support your lower back during the exercise.
- Start with shorter durations and gradually increase the time as your

strength improves.

- To exit the wall sit, slide your back up the wall, straightening your legs. Stand up and shake them out if needed.

Challenging?

- For more of a challenge, try lifting one foot slightly off the ground and holding the position on one leg, or hold a dumbbell or weighted object close to your chest to increase the intensity.

Duration

- Perform this exercise for a set duration, depending on your fitness level and workout goals.

Chair Step-Ups

A versatile exercise that can be performed almost anywhere with a stable chair or bench. They are particularly useful for strengthening the muscles involved in everyday activities such as climbing stairs and can easily be adapted by adjusting the height of the chair or bench.

Muscles engaged:

- Quadriceps and hamstrings (front and back thigh muscles)
- Glutes
- Calves
- Adductors and abductors (inner and outer thigh muscles)
- Abdominals and obliques (core muscles)
- Hip flexors (muscles at the front of the hip)

Starting Position

- Stand in front of a chair (or bench) sturdy enough to hold your weight with your feet hip-width apart.
- Keep your back straight, shoulders relaxed, and core engaged.

Begin the Exercise

- Place your right foot firmly on the chair or bench.
- Ensure your entire foot is on the surface, and your heel is not hanging off.
- Press through your right heel and lift your body onto the chair.
- Shift your weight onto your right leg as you straighten it.
- Bring your left knee up towards your chest as you stand on the chair.
- Ensure a controlled and balanced movement.
- Stand fully upright on the chair, straightening your right leg.
- Keep your left knee lifted.

Return to Starting Position

- Lower your left foot back to the ground, returning to the starting position.
- Step down with control to maintain balance.

Repetition

- Perform the same movement with your left foot on the chair, alternating between legs, for the desired number of reps.

Breathing

- Inhale as you step up.
- Exhale as you step down.

Tip on Good Form

- Focus on controlled movements to ensure proper form and reduce the risk of injury.

- Maintain a steady pace throughout the exercise, emphasizing good balance and control.
- Engage your core muscles to stabilize your torso during the movement.

Challenging?

- If you find this challenging, try reducing the height you're stepping up to, for example, using the first or second step in a set of stairs.
- For more of a challenge, after stepping up, bring your knee higher towards your chest, or hold a weighted object in each hand.

Duration

- Perform this exercise for a set duration, or a specific number of reps, depending on your fitness level and workout goals.

Single-Leg Deadlifts

A great way to target the thighs, glutes, and lower back while also improving balance and stability. They are also very effective in improving individual leg strength.

Muscles engaged:

- Quadriceps and hamstrings (front and back thigh muscles)
- Glutes
- Back muscles
- Calves
- Adductors and abductors (inner and outer thigh muscles)
- Abdominals and obliques (core muscles)

Starting Position

- Stand with your feet hip-width apart.
- Shift your weight onto one leg while keeping a slight bend in the knee.

Begin the Exercise

- Begin the movement by hinging at your hips, and pushing your hips back as you lean forward.

- Tighten your core muscles to stabilize your spine, keeping your back straight and chest lifted throughout the movement.
- Simultaneously extend the non-weight-bearing leg straight behind you.
- The extended leg and your torso should ideally form a straight line.
- Continue lowering your upper body toward the ground, reaching your hands towards the floor.
- Allow a natural bend in your standing knee, but keep it relatively stable.
- Your body should form a "T" shape, with the extended leg, torso, and arms creating parallel lines.

Return to Starting Position

- As you reach the bottom of the movement, squeeze your glutes to return to the starting position.
- Engage the muscles in your standing leg to push through the heel.

Repetition

- Complete the desired number of repetitions on one leg before switching to the other.

Breathing

- Inhale as you lower down, and exhale as you lift back up.

Tips on Good Form

- Focus on keeping your back straight, avoiding rounding or arching, and achieving a good range of motion while maintaining proper form.

- Find a focal point in front of you to help with balance.
- Engage your core to stabilize your body throughout the movement.
- Perform the exercise with a slow and controlled motion to maximize muscle engagement and reduce the risk of injury.
- Keep your weight centered over the standing foot, and avoid leaning too much to the side.
- Ensure that your standing foot is pointing forward, and the toes are not turned outward.

Challenging?

- If you find it challenging to balance, you can start with a shorter range of motion and gradually increase it as you build strength.

Duration

- Perform this exercise for a set duration, or a specific number of reps, depending on your fitness level and workout goals.

Squat Jumps

Performing squat jumps adds an explosive element to the traditional squat, combining strength and plyometric (jump) training. They are an excellent way to enhance lower body strength, power, and agility.

Muscles engaged:

- Quadriceps and hamstrings (front and back thigh muscles)
- Glutes
- Calves
- Hip flexors
- Abdominals and obliques (core muscles)
- Back muscles
- Adductors and abductors (inner and outer thigh muscles)

Start Position

- Stand with your feet shoulder-width apart.
- Keep your chest up, shoulders back, and engage your core.

Begin the Exercise

- Lower your body into a squat position by pushing your hips back and bending your knees.

- Ensure your knees stay in line with your toes, and your weight is on your heels.
- As you reach the bottom of the squat, explode upward using your leg muscles.
- Straighten your hips, knees, and ankles simultaneously, jumping off the ground.
- While in the air, extend your body fully, reaching your arms forward for balance.
- Keep your core engaged to maintain stability.
- Prepare to land by bending your knees and hips.
- Land softly on the balls of your feet, rolling through to the heels to absorb the impact.

Return to Starting Position

- After landing, immediately go back into the squat position to prepare for the next jump.
- Control the descent to engage your muscles throughout the movement.

Repetition

- Perform the squat jumps continuously, maintaining a fluid and controlled motion.
- Aim for a consistent rhythm, focusing on both the explosive upward movement and controlled landing.

Breathing

- Inhale during the squat descent and exhale explosively as you jump.

Tips on Good Form

- Keep your back straight, chest up, and knees in line with your toes during both the squat and jump phases.
- Land with a slight bend in your knees to absorb the impact and protect your joints.

Challenging?

- If you find these challenging, start with regular body weight squats (without the jump) and gradually incorporate the jumping element as your strength and comfort level increase.
- For a more intense challenge, increase the depth of your squat and the height of your jump.

Duration

- Perform this exercise for a set duration, or a specific number of reps, depending on your fitness level and workout goals.

Conclusion

While there are so many more exercises out there to choose from, this small selection can go a long way towards helping you achieve that lean, trim look. Combine the exercises however you like to create a tailor-made workout for yourself. As you progress, add in some resistance, such as weights or resistance bands to make the exercises that much more challenging. Of course, working out is only one side of the journey to getting lean – diet also plays a big part, but that is beyond the scope of this book. I hope you've found the information here useful and would appreciate it if you left a favorable review on Amazon.

Best Wishes.